Da Wu

other books in the same series

Daoyin Yangsheng Gong Shi Er Fa
12-Movement Health Qigong for all Ages
Chinese Health Qigong Association
ISBN 978 1 84819 195 2

Mawangdui Daoyin Shu
Qigong from the Mawangdui Silk Paintings
Chinese Health Qigong Association
ISBN 978 1 84819 193 8

Shi Er Duan Jin
12-Routine Sitting Exercises
Chinese Health Qigong Association
ISBN 978 1 84819 191 4

Taiji Yangsheng Zhang
Taiji Stick Qigong
Chinese Health Qigong Association
ISBN 978 1 84819 194 5

Ba Duan Jin
Eight-Section Qigong Exercises
Chinese Health Qigong Association
ISBN 978 1 84819 005 4

Yi Jin Jing
Tendon-Muscle Strengthening Qigong Exercises
Chinese Health Qigong Association
ISBN 978 1 84819 008 5

Da Wu

Health Qigong Da Wu Exercises

CHINESE HEALTH QIGONG ASSOCIATION

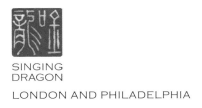

SINGING
DRAGON
LONDON AND PHILADELPHIA

This edition published in 2014
by Singing Dragon
an imprint of Jessica Kingsley Publishers
73 Collier Street
London N1 9BE, UK
and
400 Market Street, Suite 400
Philadelphia, PA 19106, USA

www.singingdragon.com

First published by Foreign Languages Press, Beijing, China, 2012

Copyright © Foreign Languages Press 2012, 2014

Library of Congress Cataloging in Publication Data
A CIP catalog record for this book is available from the Library of Congress

British Library Cataloguing in Publication Data
A CIP catalogue record for this book is available from the British Library

ISBN 978 1 84819 192 1

Printed and bound in China

CONTENTS

CHAPTER I

Origins

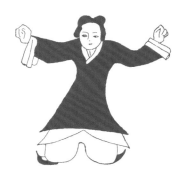

The term *Da Wu* (Da Wu Exercises) comes from the *Lu Shi* (Grand History) by Luo Mi (1131–1189) written during the Song Dynasty: "In the time of Yinkang (an ancient ruler), the ditches were not dredged and the water did not flow. It was wet and gloomy, the air was stuffy, and most people suffered from poor circulation, stiff muscles and swollen feet. So, Yinkang ordered people to dance to ease their joints, and taught people to lead the dance and convince people of its benefit. This was called the *Da Wu*."

There are also descriptions of people practicing *Da Wu* or "swelling-relieving dance" to "improve circulation" and "ease joints" in the *Shang Shu* (Book of History) compiled in the Han Dynasty. The *Huang Di Nei Jing* (Yellow Emperor's Canon of Medicine) also says: "The land in the center is flat and wet, and all things grew there. Its people ate everything and did not much labor. So most people were affected by numbness of limbs, faintness, cold and heat, and their best treatment was *daoyin* (导引) and massage."

From these descriptions, we know that "dance" was directly related to "dao (导)"; and "dance" or *Da Wu* both fall into the category of "*daoyin*" (traditional body-supporting exercise which combines breath control, body and limb movements, concentration of mind, and local massage) and have the same effect.

Apart from historical records documenting "*Da Wu*," the features and many of the movements of the dances shown in the *Pictures of Daoyin Exercises* (unearthed from the Han Dynasty tomb at Mawangdui in Changsha, Hunan Province) also provided important historical information for choreographing the Qigong *Da Wu*. Among some Stone Age tomb artifacts unearthed in Qinghai Province was a ceramic basin of the Majiayao culture of 5000 years ago, painted with vivid images of realistic dancing figures practicing ancient *qigong*. Chinese cliff paintings, murals and silk paintings from ancient times also recorded an abundance of "dancing" elements. The Zenghouyi Chimes unearthed in Suizhou of Hubei Province and the dance with its music accompaniment indicate many forms of dancing with musical accompaniment, providing an important basis for the study of the forms and characteristics of the movements of these primitive "dances." Therefore, both the written records of the *Da Wu* and the pictures of real objects of dance showed that the Chinese ancestors knew how to use the form of "dance" to relieve the pains of illness and restore health.

Choreographing the *Da Wu* as exercise today enriches the practice of *qigong* to preserve health, with an emphasis on "easing joints" and using "dancing to relieve pains through circulation." *Da Wu* uses limb movements, breath and concentration of the mind to regulate the inner organs, promote the circulation of *qi* and blood, replenish vital energy and recover from illness, thus promoting fitness.

CHAPTER II

CHARACTERISTICS

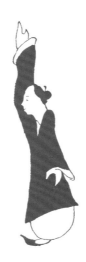

1. Dancing for Health

The *Da Wu* is based on simple dance movements of ancient times. It blends the method of *daoyin* to open up and remove obstacles to the regulation of the vital energy and functions of the human body, improves the flow of *qi* (vital energy) and blood and enhances functions of the joints.

In the movements of the body, the bones serve as levers, the joints as fulcrums, and muscle contraction provides the motor force. Each joint is a mechanism, and it moves with the internal or external changes of the body.

The main purpose of the *Da Wu* was to relax the joints and relieve pain; that is, to soften the joints, regulate and improve the meridian system (main and collateral channels), and hasten the flow of *qi* and blood to the limbs and body through the flexing and rotation of the joints at the hips, knees, toes, shoulders, elbows, wrists, palms and fingers. At the same time, the *Da Wu* uses pulling, stretching, rotating, shaking and rubbing to relieve the joints, muscles and blood vessels and the corresponding channels and to improve the circulation of *qi* and blood. Dance not only helps the muscles but also the internal organs to promote the circulation of *qi* and blood.

2. Concentrating the Mind on the Movements

According to Chinese traditional medicine, "mind" is the external expression of the functional activities of the "essence," *qi*, blood, fluids, internal organs, channels and limbs, the activities of consciousness and spirit (energy), and the controller of the life functions of the body. The *Da Wu* is expressed in the form of graceful dancing elements, and its charm, rhythmical movements, aesthetic feeling and pleasure are all closely related with the harmony between *qi* and blood, balance between *yin* and *yang*, coordination between internal and external, and the generation of a harmonious and peaceful mind. Therefore, the exercise emphasizes the use of the mind to lead the dance postures and style, the use of grace to make the dance postures pleasurable and the use of harmonious dance postures to harmonize the heart. The changes in dance posture direct the movements of the whole body and also helps promote fitness.

3. External Dancing and Internal Movement

Ancient "Da Wu" movements are soft and the rhythms are slow. This characteristic results from "internal movement" and "external dancing." "Internal movement" refers to the movements of the internal organs and channels and their regular changes. "External dancing" means that the body as an organic whole dances externally. The purpose of the dance is to integrate internal organ movement with the external dance movement for positive physiological effects.

4. Flexible Movement of the Body and the Circulation of *Qi*

"Body" refers to the body exercise and external movements, such as rising and lifting, sinking, concealing, protruding, horizontal twisting and the bending forward and backward of the body, with the spine as the pivot to drive the limbs.

"Rhythm" means regulation or internal expression, such as breathing and mind concentration. When the rhythm is combined with the movements, it produces the charm and particular nature of the *Da Wu*.

The "rhythm" of the *Da Wu* is expressed mainly in the changes of *yin* and *yang* during the movement, as well as the concentration of the mind and the circulation of *qi*. For example, the "body shaking exercise" is performed with the *Zhongjiao* acupoint as the starting point for the change of *yin* and *yang*, along with the movements of lifting up and sinking down corresponding to the lifting and sinking of the spleen and stomach.

The exercise emphasizes swinging the hips, with the hips forming the movements of "three bends." The exercise demonstrates ancient, simple and graceful dancing postures, but also drives the rotation, flexion and extension of the spine to direct qi along the Du meridian channel, thus giving more exercise to body parts which generally have less exercise in daily life. It also helps improve the channels, muscles and bones, and promote the circulation of qi and blood.

5. Combining Firmness with Softness to Regulate the Flow of *Qi*

The body is an organic whole made up of multiple tissue systems. The different systems cooperate with each other in motion. So a person's movement can be compared to perfect "dancing" as well as a "musical instrument" which produces different tunes. The *Da Wu* is graceful, relaxed, soft and slow, and improves internal firmness, for example in the movement of "Open Hips." The upper limbs move softly and slowly like willow twigs swaying in the wind, while the hips and shoulder joints move vertically and horizontally by stretching and contracting with relative strength. The whole set of movements display rhythmic motion, but also embody the traditional health-preserving ideas of combining yin and yang, firmness and softness.

Breathing movements refer to the natural regulation of the flow of *qi*. That is, the chest and abdomen expand, contract, rise and fall with changes in the pulling, rotating and stretching movements of the dance. Natural breathing leads to natural regulation of the flow of *qi*, helping to soften and massage the internal organs.

CHAPTER III

ESSENTIAL POINTS

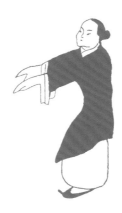

1. Relax the Mind, Hold the *Qi* and Control the Expression

In relaxing the mind, the practitioner must dispel distracting thoughts, and minimize thinking when performing the exercise. Apart from concentrating on the exercise, he or she must not have any other thoughts. Even when executing the dance movements as *daoyin*, mental activities must also be in a natural state of serene relaxation instead of purposeful consciousness. Distracting thoughts and intentional, purposeful thinking will disturb the quiet serenity of the exercise, increase the tension of the cerebral nerves and therefore reduce the health benefits.

By holding the *qi* and controlling the expression, the practitioner must concentrate on the exercise on the basis of relaxing the mind so as to achieve the integration of the body and the mind. When performing the *Da Wu*, the practitioner must remain calm and take pleasure, in an effort to achieve the harmonious integration of the graceful and pleasant dancing movements. Human emotions are closely linked with internal organs and excessive mood changes hurt them. A pleasant mood keeps the practitioner relaxed both in body and mind, and the internal *qi* soft and loose, benefiting the circulation of the blood and qi.

2. Breathe Naturally, with the *Qi* Flow Following the Movements

Natural breathing means breathing without any conscious regulation or control. There are many ways of adjusting the breath in *qigong*, but in most cases breathing is controlled by conscious awareness. The *Da Wu* requires natural breathing, however, with the rhythms of breathing determined by changes in the dancing movements. The purpose of natural breathing is to ensure the smooth flow of *qi*. This is not only good for relaxation and for coordination of movements in practicing the *Da Wu*, but is even better for relaxation of the mind. If a practitioner intentionally seeks the artistic value of the dance breathing, there will be sounds in breathing or movement of the nose. This is inconsistent with "relaxation, silence and naturalness" as advocated by the traditional thinking of health preservation, and will reduce the health benefits.

3. Combine Firmness and Softness

In practicing the *Da Wu*, a practitioner should display "firmness in softness" and "softness in firmness." The *Da Wu* places a high demand on the guided dancing movements of the limbs and harmonious movements of the body. In practicing the *Da Wu*, only when the body combines "firmness with softness" and close coordination is it possible to attain the rhythmic movements and the pleasures of harmony, lightness and flexibility for pain relief.

The Da Wu is an exercise in which dance is used to disperse and circulate pent-up qi and blood, removing obstacles from blocked channels in order to relax the joints and promote internal organ function. Therefore, when learning and practicing the Da Wu, the practitioner should attach importance both to the unblocking of the channels in the limbs, and the movement of the waist and torso. Only this awareness can fully direct the stretching and extension of the limbs and body so that movements are executed softly and fully to massage the internal organs, smooth the muscles and channels, and relax the joints to achieve overall health.

4. The Harmony of Mind and Music

The mind of the practitioner and the music must be coordinated and harmonious. The slow and melodious music helps the practitioner enter the exercise state. First the mind then the movement of the practitioner should be harmonized to the rhythms of the music. In this way, the practitioner can not only move according to the music but can also enter a state of relaxation and pleasure mode.

Slow dancing means relaxed, light, and continuous movement. At the same time, the *daoyin* of the dance must be continuous and slow. A light body and slow dance complement each other. A relaxed posture helps the *daoyin* movements look as if you are drawing an endless silk thread, and the slow-dance *daoyin* also helps the body relax. Dancing slowly with a light body also helps to relax the mind to the right state. Only when one dances with the harmony of the mind and the music and body moving with the internal rhythms, are the rise and fall, opening and closing of *qi* and blood relatively unaffected by awareness, and only then can the *daoyin* of the *Da Wu* play a better role in unblocking the channels and promoting the circulation of *qi* and blood.

CHAPTER IV

MOVEMENTS

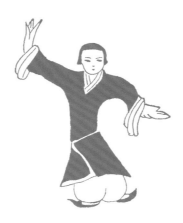

Section I Names of the Movements

Initial Stance
Step 1 Hold Head High and Chin Up (*Ang Shou Shi*)
Step 2 Open Hips (*Kai Kua Shi*)
Step 3 Extend Waist (*Chen Yao Shi*)
Step 4 Shake Body (*Zhen Ti Shi*)
Step 5 Rub Spine (*Rou Ji Shi*)
Step 6 Swing Hips (*Bai Tun Shi*)
Step 7 Massage Ribs (*Mo Lei Shi*)
Step 8 Flying Stance (*Fei Shen Shi*)
Ending Stance

Section II Movements, Tips and Health Benefits

Initial Stance

Movements

Movement 1: Place your feet together, stand with your legs naturally straight, arms at your sides, and palms lightly touching the outer legs. Tuck your chin in slightly, with your head upright, neck and back straight, chest relaxed, body erect, lips and teeth closed, tongue tip flat and lightly touching the upper jaw. Breathe naturally with a smile, eyes looking down and forward (Fig. 1).

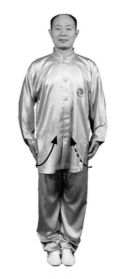

Fig. 1

Movement 2: Bend your elbows, hands held in front of the abdomen, fingers pointing to each other, palms up, and raise your hands slowly to the height of the diaphragm. Eyes are looking down and forward (Fig. 2).

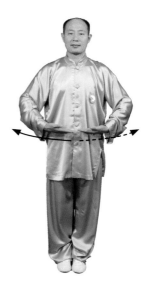

Fig. 2

Movement 3: Continue from the movement above, without pausing. Move your hands, with fingertips up and held shoulder-width apart, and turn them outward and at an angle upward and to the sides (Fig. 3). Continue the movement, lifting your arms in an arc, with both hands forward and above the forehead, arms slightly bent, palms obliquely opposite each other. Inhale with the movement, with a little pause, eyes up and forward (Fig. 4).

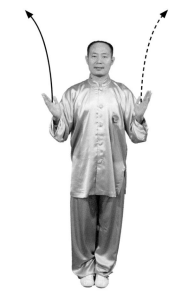

Fig. 3

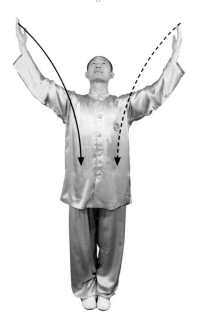

Fig. 4

Movement 4: Bend your arms, draw them inward, hands in front of your chest, fingers pointing to each other and palms facing down. Press the hands down to navel height, 10 cm apart, and draw the *qi* back to its origin. At the same time, bend your knees to about 45 degrees. Exhale, with eyes looking down and forward (Fig. 5).

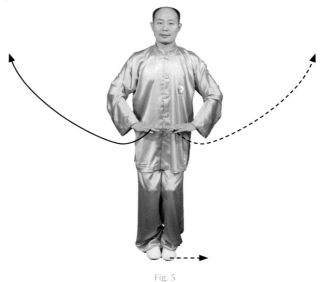

Fig. 5

Tips

1. Uplift the *Baihui* acupoint (on top of the head), keep the whole body upright and breathe naturally.

2. Relax your shoulders, relax your waist and abdomen, and tilt the sacrum down, with the anus slightly clenched.

3. *Qi* flows to the *Dantian* (lower belly). Keep calm and smile.

Health benefits

1. *Qi* flows to the *Dantian* to relieve the internal organs and relax the muscles and bones. The position promotes the circulation of *qi* and blood to get prepared for the exercise.

2. Quieten your mind. When your mind is quiet, the *qi* is held; when the *qi* is held, expression is controlled. This is good for psychological regulation.

Step 1 Hold Head High and Chin Up (*Ang Shou Shi*)
Movements

Movement 1: Continue from the initial stance. Step out with your left foot to the side, shoulder-width apart, and with knees naturally straight. At the same time, raise your arms and extend them horizontally, elbows bent slightly, palms up, fingertips lightly curved. Inhale with the movement, eyes looking forward (Fig. 6).

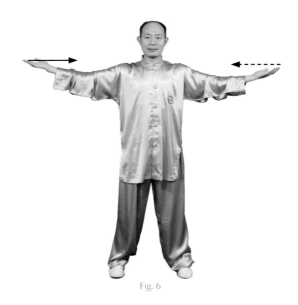

Fig. 6

Movement 2: Bend your knees to about 45 degrees and raise your head, lift your sacrum and arch your lower back. With your shoulders down and elbows dropped, wrists outward, palms up and at ear level, point your fingertips outward. Exhale with the movement, with a little pause, eyes looking up and forward (Fig. 7).

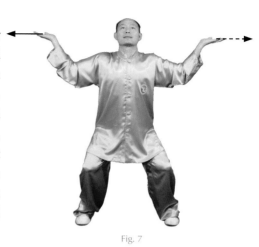

Fig. 7

Movement 3: Straighten your legs naturally, and tuck your chin in with your head upright, sacrum dropped down. Straighten your torso, extend your arms horizontally with elbows slightly bent, palms up and fingertips pointing out. Inhale with the movement, eyes looking forward (Fig. 8).

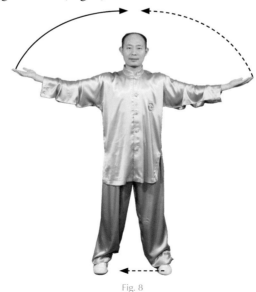

Fig. 8

Movement 4: Shift your weight to the right, move your left foot back and keep your feet together with knees straight. At the same time, raise your arms to form an arch, fingertips pointing to each other, palms obliquely down. Inhale with the movement, eyes looking forward (Fig. 9).

Then, draw the *qi* back to its origin. Move your hands in front of your chest and press them down to navel height, 10 cm apart, fingertips pointing obliquely to each other, palms down. Bend your knees at about 45 degrees and exhale with the movement, eyes looking down and ahead (Fig. 10).

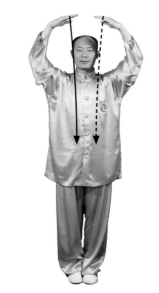

Fig. 9

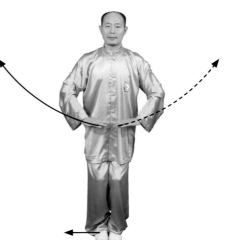

Fig. 10

Movements 5 to 8: Same as Movements 1 to 4, but move the right foot out (Figs. 11–15).

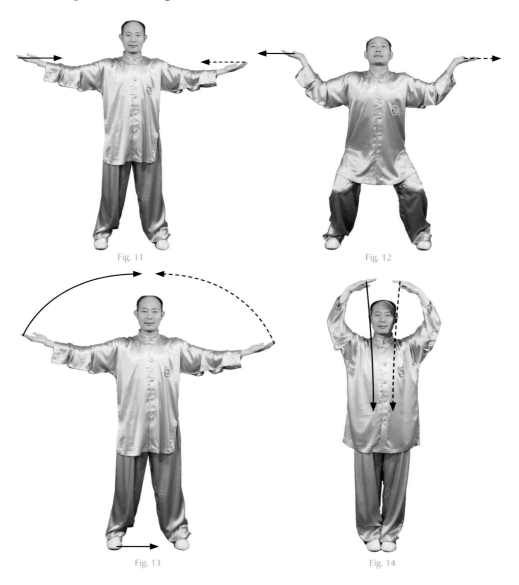

Fig. 11

Fig. 12

Fig. 13

Fig. 14

Tips

1. When squatting and arching your lower back, pull your shoulders, head and sacrum toward the *Shendao* acupoint between the shoulders, and tighten them properly. When pulling and pushing them, the shoulders are slightly forward and the head and sacrum slightly backward. When rising and standing erect, first relax your shoulders, and then the head and the sacrum.

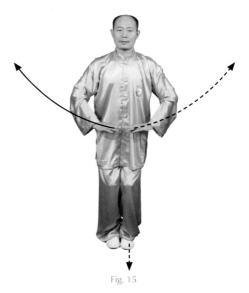

Fig. 15

2. When squatting, drop your shoulders and elbows and stretch your wrists fully.

3. When squatting and arching your back, those with back injuries should only do the exercise within their physical capacity and increase their range of motion gradually.

4. Standing up should be done slowly.

Health benefits

1. By repeatedly arching your back, you can help stretch the inter-vertebral joints.

2. By squatting and stimulating the *Shendao* acupoint, you can strengthen your legs, balance your energy, and improve the functioning of the spine, heart and lungs.

3. By arching your spine and extending your chest and abdomen, you can improve the circulation of blood in your chest and abdomen.

Step 2 Open Hips (*Kai Kua Shi*)
Movements

Movement 1: Continue from the previous movement. Shift your weight to the right, and step forward with the left foot and 30 degrees to the left to form a bow stance. At the same time, raise your arms to about 30 degrees above your head, with your palms facing each other about 20 cm apart, fingertips up and elbows bent slightly. When the arms are raised, keep the palms facing backward at first, and when your arms are raised to 45 degrees, turn them outward, with the palms gradually turned upward, and raise them above your head. Inhale with the movement, eyes looking forward (Fig. 16).

Movement 2: Continue from the previous movement. Step the right foot close to the left, sole of the foot on the ground and the heel raised, with the left knee slightly bent. At the same time, drop your shoulders and elbows, with your hands up to

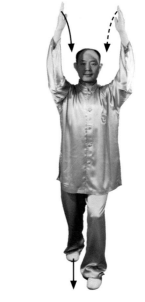

Fig. 16

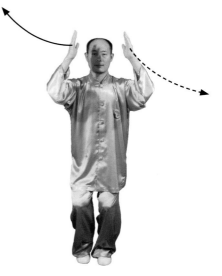

Fig. 17

about 10 cm from your forehead, palms facing each other 20 cm apart, eyes looking forward (Fig. 17).

Movement 3: Continue from the previous movement. Keep your weight on the left foot and bend the knees to 45 degrees. Swing your hips to the left, and with the sole of your right foot as the fulcrum, move your right knee outward to rotate the right leg. At the same time, spread your arms outward, the left palm at shoulder height, palm facing upward to the right, and fingertips up to the left, elbow bent slightly and the arm in an arc form. With the right palm up at 45 degrees to the right in an arc form, the palm faces the *Yuzhen* acupoint on the back of the head, fingertips up. Exhale with the movement, taking a little pause and looking at the left hand (Fig. 18 and Fig. 18 back).

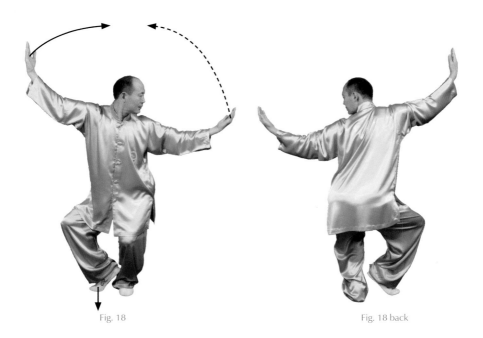

Fig. 18   Fig. 18 back

Movement 4: Straighten your left knee, and step your right foot forward and to the right to form a bow stance. At the same time, raise your arms to about 30 degrees forward and above your head, palms facing each other 20 cm apart, fingertips up, elbows slightly bent. Inhale with the movement, eyes looking forward (Fig. 19).

Movements 5 to 6: The same as Movements 2 and 3, but in the opposite direction (Fig. 20, Fig. 21 and Fig. 21 back).

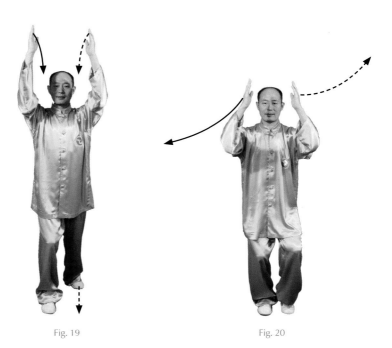

Fig. 19   Fig. 20

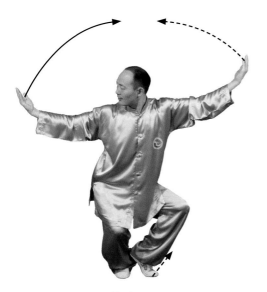

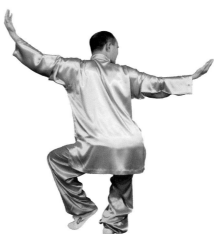

Fig. 21   Fig. 21 back

Movement 7: Straighten your right knee, and step the left foot backward 30 degrees to the left. At the same time, raise your arms to about 30 degrees forward above your head, palms facing each other, 20 cm apart, fingertips up, elbows slightly bent. Inhale with the movement, eyes forward (Fig. 22).

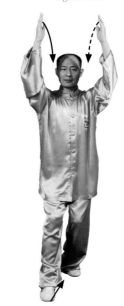

Fig. 22

Movement 8: Step your right foot back alongside the left, sole on the ground, and heel raised, with the left knee slightly bent. At the same time, drop your shoulders and elbows, and move both hands downward to 10 cm from your forehead, palms facing each other about 20 cm apart, fingertips up, eyes looking forward (Fig. 23).

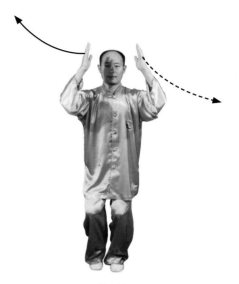

Fig. 23

Movement 9: Bend your left knee to squat at about 45 degrees. Swing your hips to the left and with the sole of the right foot as the pivot, move the right knee and rotate the right leg outward to open the right hip. Spread your arms and extend them outward, the left hand at shoulder height, palm facing up to the right, and fingertips up to the left, with the elbow bent slightly and your arm in an arc, the right palm up 45 degrees to the right, palm facing the *Yuzhen* acupoint on the back of the head, and the fingertips up. Exhale with the movement, with a little pause, eyes on the left hand (Fig. 24 and Fig. 24 back).

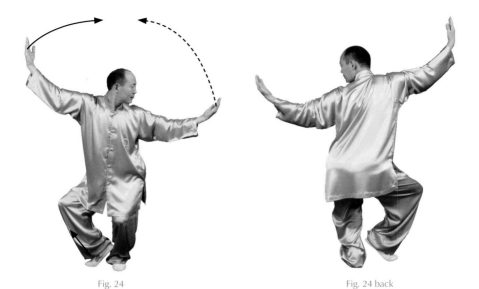

Fig. 24   Fig. 24 back

Movements 10 to 12: The same as Movements 7 to 9, but in the
opposite direction (Fig. 25, Fig. 26, Fig. 27 and Fig. 27 back).

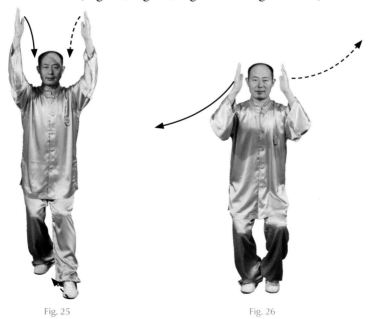

Fig. 25   Fig. 26

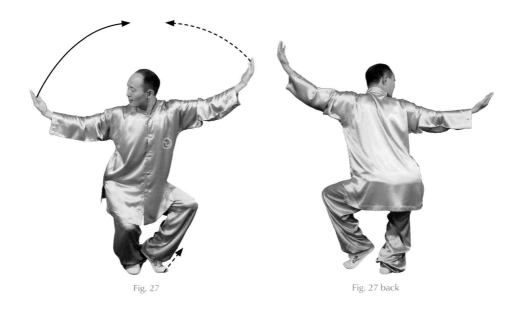

Fig. 27   Fig. 27 back

Do the open hips exercise in both directions, once with an initial forward step, and once with an initial backward step.

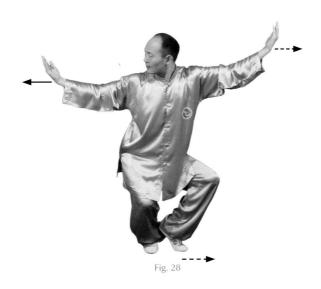

Fig. 28

Movement 13: Continuing from the backward step with open hips (Fig. 28), shift your weight to the right foot, step your left foot apart so your feet are parallel and slightly further apart than shoulder-width, with knees naturally straight. At the same time, extend your arms horizontally, elbows bent slightly, palms facing up and fingertips outward, eyes looking forward (Fig. 29).

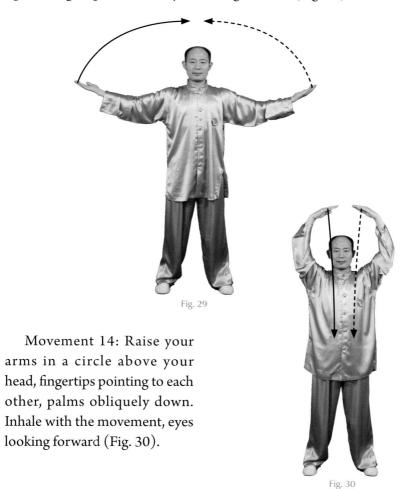

Fig. 29

Movement 14: Raise your arms in a circle above your head, fingertips pointing to each other, palms obliquely down. Inhale with the movement, eyes looking forward (Fig. 30).

Fig. 30

Movement 15: Relax the shoulders and drop your elbows, then draw the *qi* back to its origin. Press your palms downward to navel level in front of your abdomen, 10 cm apart, fingertips pointing to each other. At the same time, bend your knees at about 45 degrees. Exhale with the movement, eyes looking down and forward (Fig. 31).

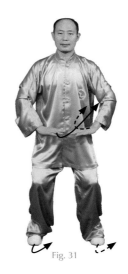

Fig. 31

Tips

1. When swinging the hips, the opposite leg should be rotated outward fully, and stretched left and right.

2. When the arms are spread, your shoulder blades should be pulled outwards to the sides. At the same time, turn your head on the level.

3. When swinging the hips, use your ribcage to draw the swinging, pulling the caudal vertebrae and cervical vertebrae one by one. There should be "softness with firmness" in the movement.

4. Both the forward step and backward step should be steady, and the movements should be executed slowly.

5. When the spine is flexed and extended sideways, the execution of the movements will vary from person to person depending on your flexibility.

Health benefits

1. By opening, closing and rotating to pull and extend the shoulders and hips, the exercise helps to use the big joints to drive the small joints.

2. By flexing and extending the shoulders and arms through the spine when opening the hips, extend the arms to the sides to draw the ribs, with the *Dadun* acupoint on the side of the big toe touching the ground to turn outward. This restores the normal flow of liver *qi* and promotes the flow of *qi* and blood, as well as increases the strength of the legs and improves their balance.

Step 3 Extend Waist (*Chen Yao Shi*)

Movements

Movement 1: Continue from the previous movement. Shift your weight to the left, turn your right foot inward and shift your weight back to the right with the left heel as the pivot, toes turned outward about 90 degrees and body turned 90 degrees to the left. At the same time, put your hands together by your diaphragm and raise them slightly, 20 cm between your joined palms and chest, toes up and forward, eyes looking forward (Fig. 32).

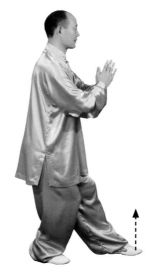

Fig. 32

Movement 2: Straighten the right leg and raise your left knee, calf relaxed and toes pointing down and inward. Keep your wrists at the same height as the *Tanzhong* acupoint at the middle of the chest, about 10 cm from chest. Fingertips point forward, about 30 degrees from the vertical line, eyes looking forward (Fig. 33).

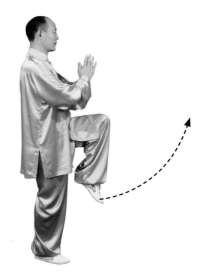

Fig. 33

Movement 3: Straighten the right leg, and kick the left foot out straight in front, toes turned up, eyes looking forward (Fig. 34).

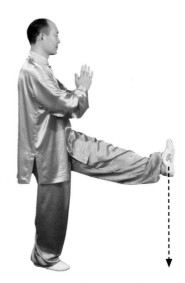

Fig. 34

Movement 4: Bend the right knee and step forward with the left foot, 30 degrees to the left to form a bow stance, eyes looking forward (Fig. 35).

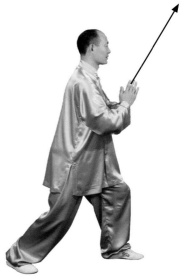

Fig. 35

Movement 5: With your feet on the ground, bend the torso forward 45 degrees, extending your hands forward and upward, eyes looking up and forward. When your arms are straight, tuck in your chin, turning your eyes down and forward. Then extend your arms forward with your upper arms against your ears and push the right heel down and backward. Inhale with the movement, taking a little pause (Fig. 36).

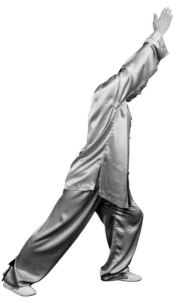

Fig. 36

Movement 6: Keeping the left foot in place, raise your right heel with the right toes grasping the ground. Continue to extend the arms forward and upward. Inhale with the movement, with a little pause, eyes looking down and forward (Fig. 37).

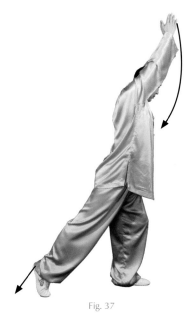

Fig. 37

Movement 7: Shift your weight backward and plant your right heel on the ground, with the right knee deeply bent. At the same time, turn the sole and toes of the left foot up, straighten your left leg, hips up, waist down and chest out. Move the hands back to the *Danzhong* acupoint, about 15 cm from your chest, fingertips up and angled 30 degrees forward from the vertical line. Exhale with the movement, with a little pause, eyes looking up and forward (Fig. 38).

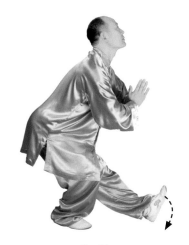

Fig. 38

Movements 8 to 13: Repeat Movements 2 to 7.

Movement 14: Continue from the previous movement. Rise, bend your right leg slightly, with the sole of the left foot turned sharply inward (Fig. 39). Shift your weight to the left, extend the right toes sharply outward and turn 180 degrees to the right, eyes looking directly ahead (Fig. 40).

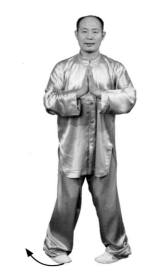

Fig. 39

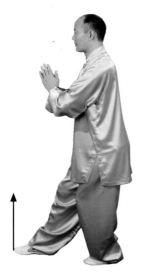

Fig. 40

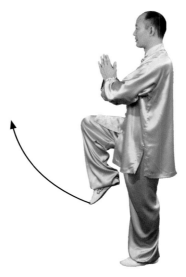

Fig. 41

Repeat Movements 2 to 7 twice in the opposite direction (Figs. 41–46).

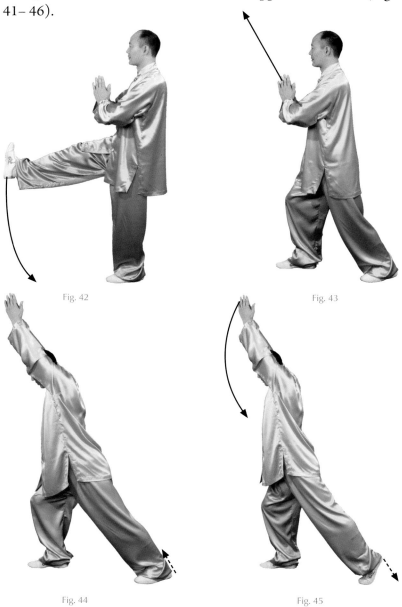

Fig. 42

Fig. 43

Fig. 44

Fig. 45

In this exercise, one forward extension and one shift backward constitute a routine; first do two routines to the left and then two routines to the right.

Movement 15: Straighten your left leg and rise, the sole of the right foot turned inward about 90 degrees, toes forward. Shift your weight to the right, twist your left heel inward about 45 degrees, keep your feet parallel at shoulder-width, and stand erect, eyes looking forward (Fig. 47). Then bend the knees about 45 degrees, move your hands apart and turn them down, fingertips pointing obliquely to each other. Press the palms down to the height of the navel, 10 cm from the abdomen, with the *qi* drawn back to its origin. Exhale with the movement, eyes looking down and forward (Fig. 48).

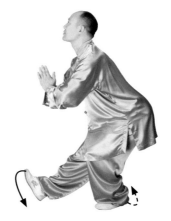

Fig. 46

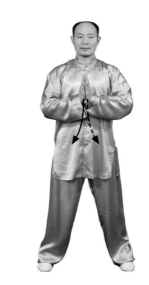

Fig. 47

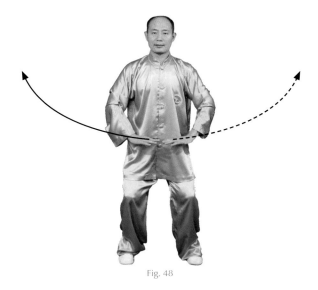

Fig. 48

Tips

1. When stretching forward, push your hands up and press down with your rear foot.

2. When stretching forward, your arms, body and rear leg should form a straight line.

3. When your weight is shifting backward, turn the big toe of the front foot upward at the *Dadun* acupoint on the outside of the toe. At the same time, thrust out the thehips and lower your waist fully.

4. When you step forward, avoid placing your feet in a straight line, and keep your body steady.

5. When stretching forward, make sure to avoid using sudden or rigid force. There should be "tightness in relaxation." Do the stretching movements slowly and softly.

6. When the palms are put together, leave a hollow between them.

Health benefits

When stretching your hands and feet slowly forward, the joints and tendons will also be stretched with the *Du* and *Sanjiao* meridian channels opened for better circulation of the *qi* and blood in the muscles, tendons and soft tissues around joints.

By arching the lower back, turning the tail up, thrusting the chest, raising the head, putting your palms together and drawing them in front of the *Tanzhong* acupoint, you can help regulate the circulation along the *Ren* and *Du* meridian channels and the function of the heart and lungs. By drawing and pulling the spine in opposite directions, you improve the flexibility of your upper back as well as the leg joints.

Step 4 Shake Body (*Zhen Ti Shi*)

Movements

Movement 1: Continue from the previous movement. Straighten your legs and raise your arms to extend them horizontally, palms down, fingertips outward. Inhale with the movement, eyes looking forward (Fig. 49).

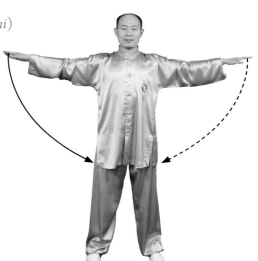

Fig. 49

Movement 2: Bend your knees and widen yours stance as if riding a horse. Drop your arms to about 45 degrees, bend the elbows and move your arms back in an arc to shoulder-width, the upper arms down at about 45 degrees forward, to the height of the navel, palms up and fingertips forward. Exhale with the movement, eyes looking at the palms (Fig. 50).

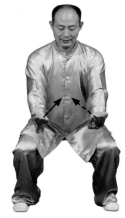

Fig. 50

Movement 3: Straighten the legs slowly and clench your fists tightly, with the thumbs just touching the inner sides of the ring fingers, and doubling the other fingers one by one. Place them in front of the abdomen, fists facing each other and fingers up, lightly touching the sides of the navel, eyes looking forward (Fig. 51).

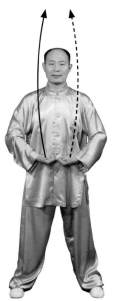

Fig. 51

Then shift your weight to the right, bend the left knee and raise it higher than level, calf down and toes up. Turn your forearms inward until the fist backs are opposite to each other, about five cm apart, wrists raised naturally. Move hands above your head, elbows bent slightly, fists facing each other, about 10 cm apart. Inhale with the movement, eyes looking forward (Fig. 52).

Movement 4: Relax your left leg and swing it down and backward about 15 degrees from the vertical line, relaxing your shoulders and dropping your elbows, arms hanging naturally, and relax your fists when the arms are moved down, palms up and fingertips outward. Continue the movement, rotate the arms inward and downward, with the *Hegu* acupoints on the hands lightly touching the *Dan* meridian channel at the middle of the outer thigh. Exhale with the movement, eyes looking forward (Fig. 53).

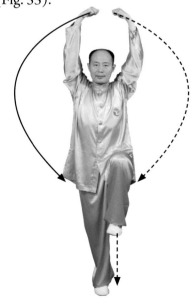
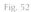

Fig. 52

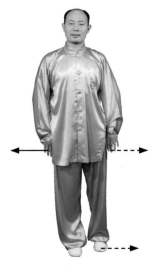

Fig. 53

Step your left foot to the left, with the feet apart slightly wider than shoulder-width. Plant the feet, big toes first and then heels, and straighten your legs naturally. At the same time, raise both arms to 45 degrees (Fig. 54).

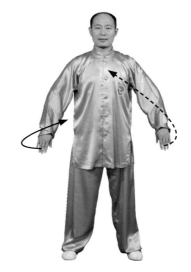

Fig. 54

Movement 5: Turn your body 45 degrees to the right, with the left hand moving in an arc to the midline in front of the body at the same height as the *Tanzhong* acupoint, palm up with the fingers bent. When drawing the arc, turn the left arm gradually outward, elbow bent slightly. At the same time, move the right hand to draw an arc to the midline behind the body at the same height as the *Mingmen* acupoint on the lower back, palm up with the fingers bent (when drawing the arc, turn the right arm gradually inward, elbow slightly bent). Inhale with the movement, eyes looking at the left hand (Fig.55 and Fig. 55 back).

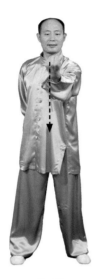

Fig. 55

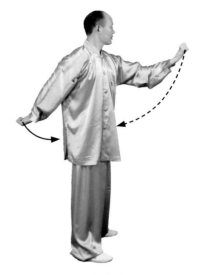

Fig. 55 back

Movement 6: Bend slightly at the knees, turning the body back to the front. Relax your shoulders and drop the elbows, with the ulnar side of the left fist touching the lower *Dantian* lightly, and the radial side of the right fist touching the sacrum lightly. Exhale with the motion, eyes looking down forward (Fig. 56).

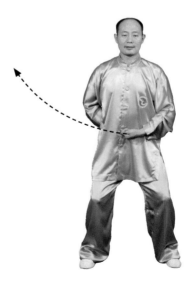

Fig. 56

Movement 7: Straighten the legs slowly and turn your torso 90 degrees to the right, relax your fists, extend the left hand to the right, elbow bent slightly, palm up at the same height as the *Tanzhong* acupoint, fingertips to the right; extend the right hand to the left, elbow bent slightly, palm up at the same height as the *Mingmen* acupoint, fingertips to the left, looking at the left hand (Fig. 57). Then, turn back to the front to drive the left hand to move from the right forward, forward, to the left forward, and the right hand to move from the left backward, backward, to the right backward in an arc to the right, finishing with your arms extending horizontally, elbows bent slightly, palms facing the ground, fingertips pointing outward, eyes looking forward (Fig. 58).

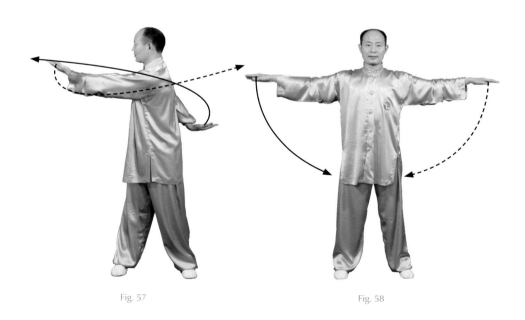

Fig. 57   Fig. 58

Movements 8 to 13: The same as Movements 2 to 7, but in the opposite direction (Figs. 59–66). Then repeat Movements 2 to 13, once to the right and once to the left per routine. Do the routine twice.

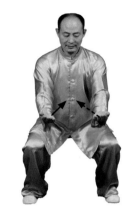

Fig. 59

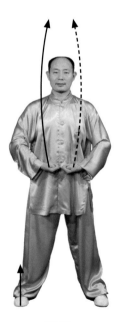

Fig. 60

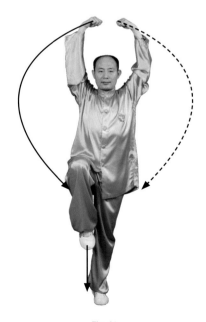

Fig. 61

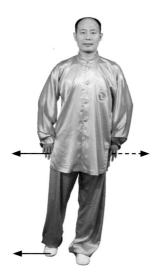

Fig. 62

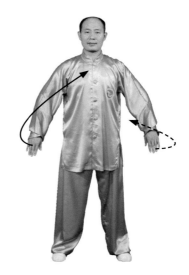

Fig. 63

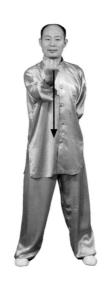

Fig. 64

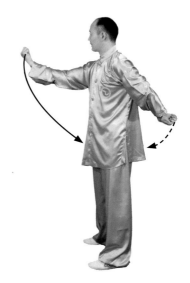

Fig. 64 back

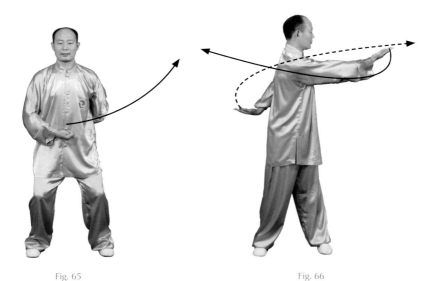

Fig. 65   Fig. 66

Continue from the previous finish (Fig. 67). Straighten your legs slowly, relaxing your fists, with the left hand moving downward to the left and upward, and the right hand moving downward to the right and upward to form a circle, with your fingertips pointing to each other and palms down. Inhale with the movement, eyes looking forward (Fig. 68).

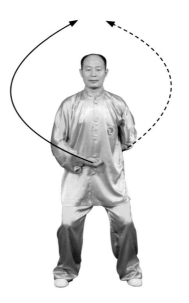

Fig. 67

Then, bend the legs about 45 degrees, and press your palms downward, to the level of your navel in front of the abdomen, 10 cm apart, with the *qi* drawn back to the origin, fingertips pointing obliquely to each other. Exhale, eyes looking down and forward (Fig. 69).

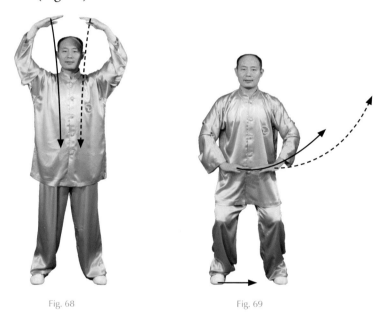

Fig. 68   Fig. 69

Tips

1. Sequence the motions from above to below in raising the knee and the clenched fist. When moving the leg downward, relax. The power originates from the momentum of the movements.

2. When raising the knees or arms, inhale with the motion, and extend the waist upward at the same time.

3. Relax your shoulders, drop the elbows and draw the wrists when your arm touches the *Qihai* meridian channel and sacrum

at the same time, with the power coming from the momentum of dropping your arms.

4. The height of the raised knee varies from person to person.

5. The movements should be light and slow when swinging the leg.

Health benefits

1. Increase the flexibility of the waist by turning the *Dai* meridian channel and spine. Beat the *Dan* meridian channel to shake the *Dantian*, muster the genuine energy, and support the primordial energy so that the *qi* is directed, the muscles are nourished and the blood is circulated to increase your ability to resist illness.

2. Execute the movement of passive traction through the inertia of the torso and limbs arising from the practitioner's own weight. Extend the joints to pull the joints of the hips and knees to relieve the damage caused by chronic overload. It helps to keep the leg joints in good shape or helps them to recover.

Step 5 Rub Spine (*Rou Ji Shi*)
Movements

Movement 1: Continue from the previous movement. Shift your weight to the left and move the right foot back in line with the left, the sole of the right foot on the ground and the heel raised. At the same time, your arms flow downward, then to the left and upward to shoulder height, palms down and fingertips extended, with the right arm at about 45 degrees relative to the left, and fingertips also pointing left. Bend both elbows slightly and inhale with the movement, eyes looking at the left hand (Fig. 70).

Movement 2: Continue the movement. Keep your left leg bent at 45 degrees, and with the sole of your right foot as the pivot, drive the right leg to twist outward till the toes are pointed left. At the same time, swing your hips to the left and bend your torso to the right at about 45 degrees from vertical line. Drive the left arm far upward to the right, about 45 degrees from vertical line, with the elbow bent slightly, palm up and fingertips pointed right. Move the right hand beneath the left armpit, with the *Laogong* acupoint on the right hand at the same height as the *Dabao* acupoint on the lateral side of the chest, 10 cm apart, the elbow bent. Inhale with the movement, eyes following the left hand. When the trunk is bent about 45 degrees to the right, turn the head to the right. Inhale with the movement, adding a short pause, eyes looking down and to the right (Fig. 71).

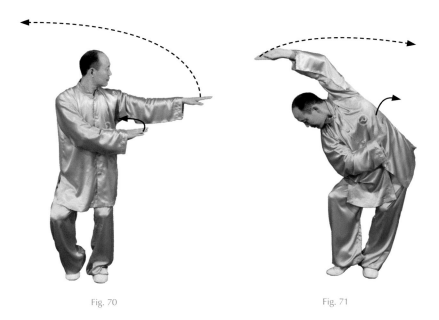

Fig. 70   Fig. 71

Movement 3: Start from the concluding form of Movement 2 and return to Movement 1 along the original route of the movement (Fig. 72).

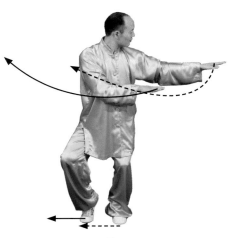

Fig. 72

Movement 4: Step the right foot out to the right, with the feet apart slightly wider than shoulder-width, shift your weight to the right, with the right knee slightly bent. Move your left foot back in line with the right, left sole on the ground and heel raised. At the same time, move the arms downward and swing them to the right, the right arm to the height of the shoulder, palm down and fingertips to the right, and the left arm beneath it, about 45 degrees from vertical line. Both elbows are bent slightly, palms down, fingertips outward. Inhale with the movement, eyes looking at the right hand (Fig. 73).

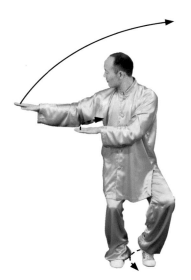

Fig. 73

Movement 5: The same as Movement 2, but in the opposite direction (Fig. 74 and Fig. 74 back).

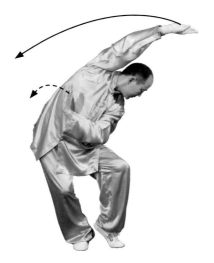

Fig. 74

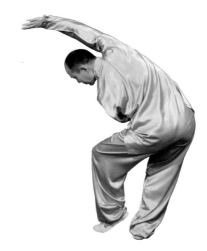

Fig. 74 back

Movement 6: Start from the final position of Movement 5 and return to Movement 4 along the original route of the movement (Fig. 75).

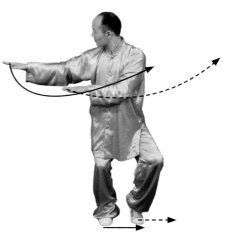

Fig. 75

Movement 7: The same as Movement 4, but in the opposite direction (Fig. 76).

Repeat Movements 2 to 6.

This sequence is done once to the right and once to the left in a routine. Do the whole routine twice.

Continue from the last movement (Fig. 77). Step out with the left foot, and set your feet parallel and slightly wider than shoulder-width, with legs straight. At the same time, drop your arms to shoulder level, outstretched with elbows bent slightly, palms up and fingertips pointing outward (Fig. 78).

Then raise your arms to form a circle, fingertips pointing at each other, 10 cm apart, with palms down and arms in an arc. Inhale with the movement, eyes looking forward (Fig. 79).

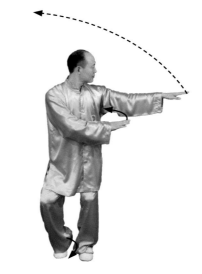

Fig. 76

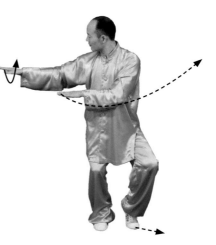

Fig. 77

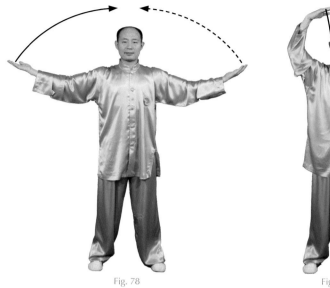

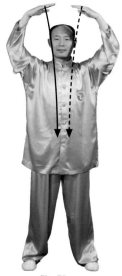

Fig. 78   Fig. 79

Then, bend the knees to 45 degrees and draw the *qi* back to the origin. Press the hands down to the navel level in front of your abdomen, about 10 cm apart, with fingertips pointing obliquely to each other. Exhale with the movement, eyes looking down and forward (Fig. 80).

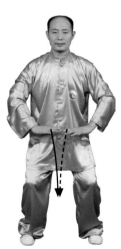

Fig. 80

Tips

1. When starting or finishing foot movement, the movements should be light. When drawing your hips back and raising the knees, use your waist.

2. When turning or swinging the arms to the right or left and above, the movements from the waist to the chest and from the shoulders to the hands should be soft, slow and flowing.

3. Match the movements with your breathing. Inhale when raising your arms and exhale when lowering them.

4. Move your feet steadily; the range of motion varies from person to person.

5. Perform the movements one after another without pause.

Health benefits

1. Sideways bending and extension of the spine help enhance the elasticity of the ligaments and the strength of the muscles supporting the spine.

2. Sideways bending and extension of the spine and rotation of the legs outward help to restore the normal flow of liver *qi* and ventilate the lung *qi*.

Step 6 Swing Hips (*Bai Tun Shi*)
Movements

Movement 1: Continue from the previous movement. Bend your legs to 45 degrees, and hold the bend, tucking the chin in and facing down. Extend and bend slowly, from top to bottom and one by one, the cervical vertebra, thoracic vertebra, lumbar vertebra and sacrum and the spinal segments, to 45 degrees forward. At the same time, press your palms together along the vertical line between your knees, gradually turning the fingertips down, with the backs of your hands against each other, and elbows bent slightly, eyes looking at the hands (Fig. 81).

Movement 2: Straighten your legs slowly and stand erect, after straightening the spinal segments and the head, one by one and from bottom to top. Raise your arms simultaneously, keep your forearms at the same level to place your palms together at chest level, fingertips

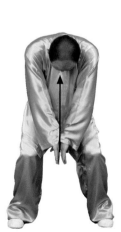

Fig. 81

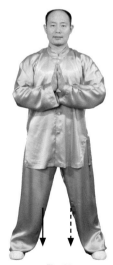

Fig. 82

pointed down. Continue the movement, relax your shoulders and drop the elbows, and gradually turn your fingertips up and keep your palms together in front of your chest, with forearms and palms at the same height as the *Tanzhong* acupoint, about 10 cm apart. Inhale with the movement, eyes looking down and forward (Fig. 82)

Movement 3: Bend your knees at 45 degrees, and execute the following movements the same as above (Fig. 83).

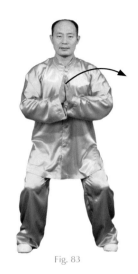

Fig. 83

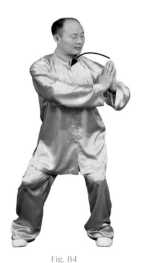

Fig. 84

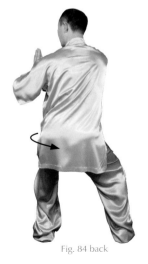

Fig. 84 back

Movement 4: With your knees and toes in the same direction, head upright and neck straight, shift your hips to the left and forward slowly. At the same time, push your joined hands to the left and forward slowly. Inhale with the movement, take a little pause, eyes looking down and toward the left (Fig. 84 and Fig. 84 back).

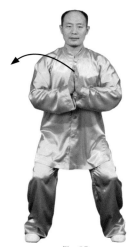

Fig. 85

Movement 5: Relax the hips and arms, return to the original position, execute just like Movement 3 (Fig. 85).

Movement 6: The same as Movement 4, but in the opposite direction (Fig. 86 and Fig. 86 back).

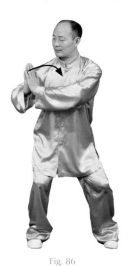

Fig. 86

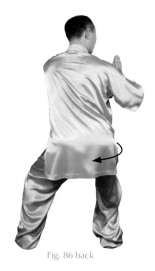

Fig. 86 back

Movement 7: Relax the hips and arms, return to the original position, and execute in the same way as Movement 3 (Fig. 87).

Repeat Movements 4 to 7.

Movement 8: With your knees and toes in the same direction, head upright and neck straight, swing your hips to the left. At the same time, bend your joined hands 45 degrees leftward at the wrists, eyes looking down and forward on the left side (Fig. 88 and Fig. 88 back). Continue the movement.

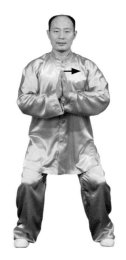

Fig. 87

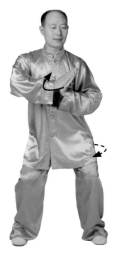

Fig. 88

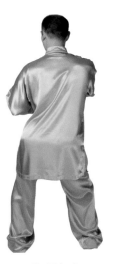

Fig. 88 back

With the sacrum as the center, turn in a clockwise circle twice. At the same time, with the wrists as the axis and the middle fingertips as the point, draw a flat circle clockwise twice. When drawing the circle with the hands, keep a 45-degree angle from the vertical line. Breathe naturally, eyes following the circle you are drawing. Continue the movement at the conclusion of the second circle, and move the sacrum and hands forward; return them to the original position in an arc (Fig. 89).

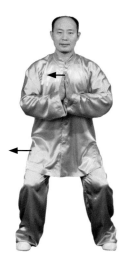

Fig. 89

Movement 9: The same as Movement 8, but in the opposite direction (Fig. 90, Fig. 90 back and Fig. 91).

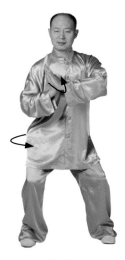 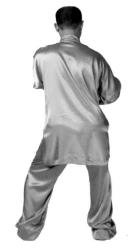

Fig. 90   Fig. 90 back

This exercise is done once to the right and then once to the left in a routine. Repeat it in each direction. Then, draw two circles clockwise and two circles counterclockwise.

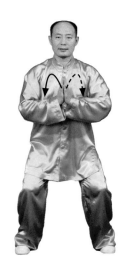

Fig. 91

Movement 10: As you finish the second counterclockwise circle, separate your fingers, from the thumb to the little finger one by one in order, turn your palms up and fingertips forward (Fig. 92). Then, join your fingers from the little finger to the thumb in order and turning your wrists, thrust your hands backward from beneath your armpits to your back, just below the shoulder blades, palms facing backward, fingertips down, and wrist joints touching the sides of the spine (Fig. 93 and Fig. 93 back).

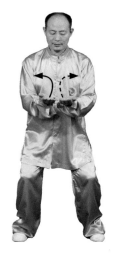

Fig. 92

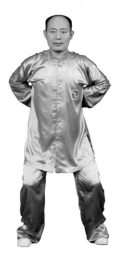

Fig. 93

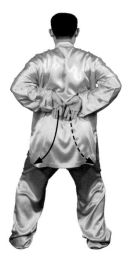

Fig. 93 back

Movement 11: Straighten your legs slowly. At the same time, press the hands downward to the *Huantiao* acupoint at the top of the hips. Inhale with the movement, eyes looking forward (Fig. 94 and Fig. 94 back).

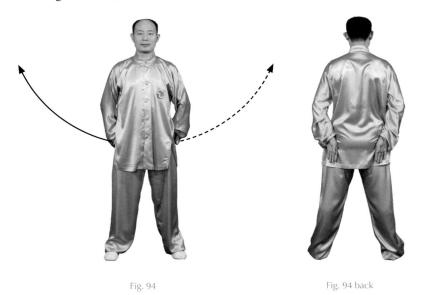

Fig. 94   Fig. 94 back

Then, turn your arms gradually outward, raise them, and extend them horizontally (Fig. 95). Continue this movement, and lift them up to form a circle, fingertips pointing to each other about 10 cm apart, with your eyes looking forward (Fig. 96).

Next, bend your knees 45 degrees. At the same time, draw the *qi* back to its origin, move your hands in front of the body and press them downward to navel height, about 10 cm apart, with fingertips obliquely pointing to each other, palms down. Inhale with the movement, eyes looking down and forward (Fig. 97).

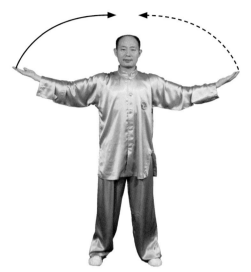

Fig. 95

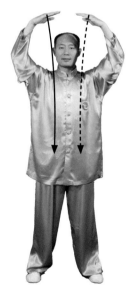

Fig. 96

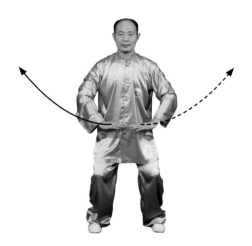

Fig. 97

Tips

1. When swinging your hips to the left or right, with the sacrum as the focal point, swing your waist and chest softly and slowly with the help of your hip movement, without shifting your weight in any direction.

2. Move your hands and sacrum in the same direction, with your eyes following the movement of the hands, looking down and forward.

3. Don't pull forcefully when swinging the hips.

4. Your range of movement should grow from light to strong. Don't do it beyond your ability.

5. When putting your palms together, keep a hollow between them.

Health benefits

1. In swinging the hips, use your sacrum to drive the movement of the spine and limbs. This produces a massaging effect on the spine and internal organs. It can relieve the internal organs and increase the flexibility of the waist and hips.

2. Turning with the palms together can help push, massage, draw and pull the joints of the shoulders, elbows, wrists and fingers.

3. The regulation of the *Ren*, *Chong* and *Dai* meridian channels helps relieve the strains on the muscles of the legs and lower back.

Step 7 Massage Ribs (*Mo Lei Shi*)
Movements

Movement 1: Continue from the previous movement. Straighten your legs, raise your arms and extend them horizontally, palms down and fingertips outward. Inhale with the motion, eyes looking forward (Fig. 98).

Movement 2: Shift your weight to the right, pivot the sole of the left foot 45 degrees inward, and then shift your weight to the left, with your left leg bent slightly and your right leg straight, with the toes of the right foot turned up. Using the right heel as the fulcrum, rotate the foot 90 degrees. At the same time, turn the body about 90 degrees to the right (Fig. 99). Continue the movement, shift your weight back, and bend forward to drive the arms to draw circles: move the left arm upward, forward and downward until the

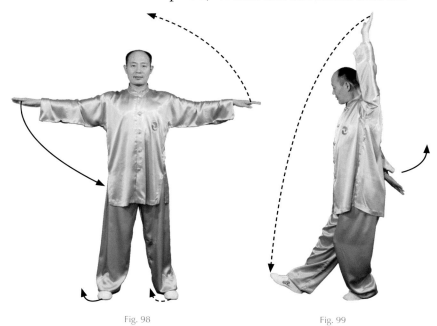

Fig. 98   Fig. 99

left palm lightly touches the right toes, fingertips pointing forward and elbow bent slightly. At the same time, move your right arm downward, backward and upward to extend horizontally backward, palm up, and fingertips pointing back and up, with your elbow bent slightly. Exhale with the movement, taking a little pause, with your eyes looking down and forward (Fig. 100 and Fig. 100 back).

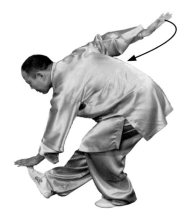 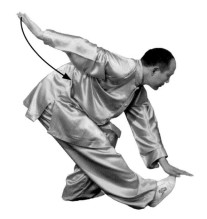

Fig. 100   Fig. 100 back

Movement 3: Bend the right elbow, and place your right palm on your ribs just above your waist (Fig. 101). Next, stand erect and immediately turn to the left, push and rub the base of the right palm downward along the sideline of the torso to the area below

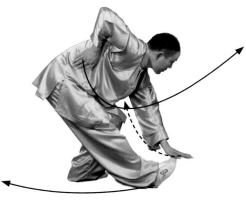

Fig. 101

the hip. Then move your right hand forward to draw an arc upward and forward to the midline at the height of the *Tanzhong* acupoint, right elbow bent slightly, palm down and fingertips pointed forward. Then move the left hand upward in an arc from the outer left hip to the ribcage beneath your left armpit, palm inward and fingertips down. Exhale with the movement, eyes looking at the right hand (Fig. 102).

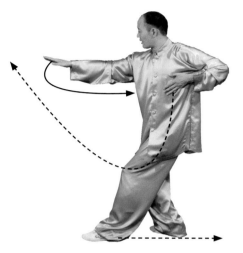

Fig. 102

Movement 4: Move the left foot back about 30 degrees to the left, shifting your weight backwards to leave your right foot unweighted. At the same time, turn your torso to the right, push and rub the base of the left palm downward along the sideline of your ribs to the area below your hip. Then swing your left hand forward to draw an arc upward to the midline at the height of the *Tanzhong* acupoint, left elbow bent slightly, palm facing down and fingertips forward. At the same time, move the right hand upward in an arc along the outer side of the right hip to just beneath the right armpit, palm inward and fingertips down. Exhale with the movement, eyes focused on the left hand (Fig. 103).

Movement 5: The same as Movement 4, but in the opposite direction (Fig. 104).

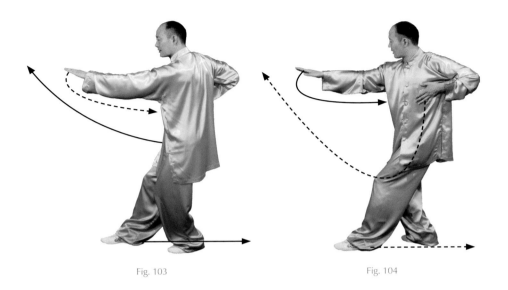

Fig. 103   Fig. 104

Movement 6: The same as Movement 4 (Fig. 103).

Movement 7: Continue from the fourth movement of rib massage with a backward step (Fig. 105). Bend the weighted left leg, and keep the right leg straight, with toes turned up, shifting your weight backward and bending your torso forward at the same time. Press the left palm downward, lightly touching the right toes, with fingertips pointing forward. Move the right arm downward, past the outside of the right hip in an arc up and backward, extending the arm, palm up and fingertips up pointing backward. Exhale with the movement, and add a little pause, eyes looking down and forward (Fig. 106).

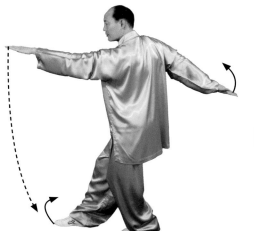

Fig. 105

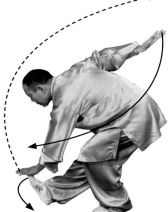

Fig. 106

Movement 8: Rise up, with the sole of the right foot turned inward 135 degrees. Continue the movement, shifting your weight to the right, with the left foot turned outward 135 degrees and toes turned up. Straighten your left leg and turn 180 degrees to the left.

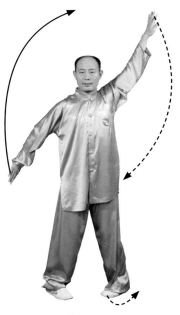

Fig. 107

Continue the motion, shift your weight backward and bend your torso forward to turn the left arm inward, forward, and upward, past the head, then down and backward and extended up, palm and fingertips up pointing backward, elbow bent slightly; turn the right arm downward, upward, past the head, then forward, and extended down, palm slightly touching the left toes and fingertips pointing forward. Exhale with the movement, with a little pause, eyes looking down and forward (Figs. 107–109).

Movements 9 to 13: Repeat Movements 3 to 7, but on the opposite side (Figs. 110–115).

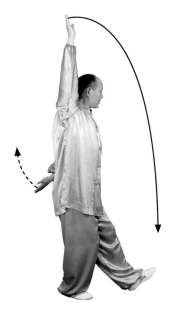

Fig. 108

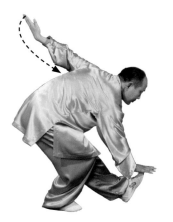

Fig. 109

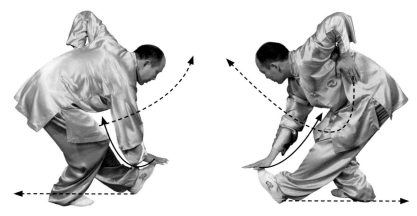

Fig. 110   Fig. 110 back

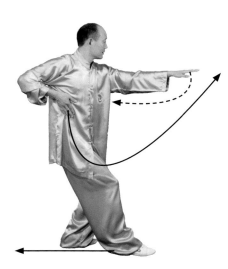

Fig. 111

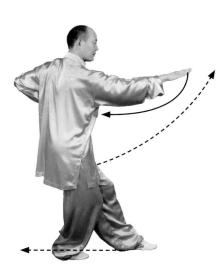

Fig. 112

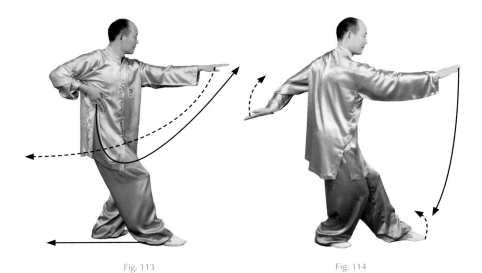

Fig. 113   Fig. 114

In this position, move back four steps on the left side and massage your left-side ribs four times, then move back four steps on the right side and massage your ribs four times on the right. So, massage your ribs four times per routine and execute the routine in both left and right directions.

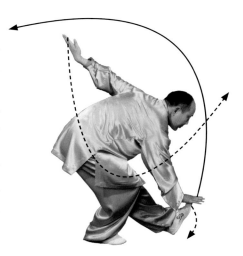

Fig. 115

Movement 14: Continue from the end of Movement 13 (Fig. 115). Turn the sole of the left foot inward, toes forward, shifting your weight slightly to the left, with the right heel pivoting inward 45 degrees, feet positioned at shoulder-width; and straighten your legs. At the same time, rise up and turn your body 90 degrees to the right, body upright, turn the left arm inward and forward, upward and past the head; then extend it to the right side, palm up and fingertips outward. Move the left arm downward, and upward from the left and extend it horizontally to the left side, palm up and fingertips outward, eyes looking forward (Fig. 116).

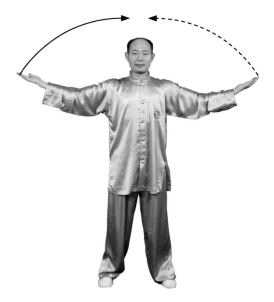

Fig. 116

Now raise your arms to form a circle, fingertips pointing to each other, 10 cm apart, palms obliquely facing down. Inhale with the motion, eyes looking ahead (Fig. 117).

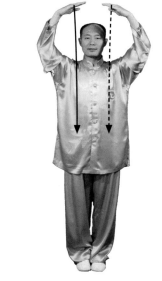

Fig. 117

Then, bend the legs about 45 degrees and draw the *qi* back to the origin. Move the palms in front of your body and press them down to waist level, 10 cm apart, fingertips obliquely pointing to each other and palms down. Exhale with the movement, eyes looking down forward (Fig. 118).

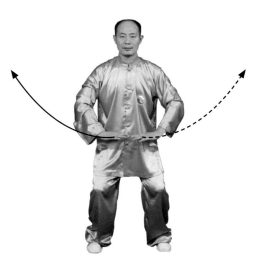

Fig. 118

1. Use your waist to drive the spine in turning your body to the right or left. At the same time, beginning from the *Dabao* acupoint, use the heel of your hand to massage your ribs downward from the armpit along the sideline of the body. The ribs should be pressed and massaged one by one smoothly and continuously, with the eyes following the movement of the hands. Do the exercise calmly.

2. When massaging your ribs, use the *qi* from the lower *Dantian* to move the waist, use your waist to drive the shoulders, use your shoulders to drive the arms and use your arms to drive the wrists, and extend to fingertips, to use the *qi* to relieve the internal organs and then to relax your joints.

3. This exercise requires a high degree of coordination, and practicing the movements that are hard to coordinate helps to improve your performance.

4. For beginners, a movement can be separated into parts. For example, first practice the backward step, then massage the ribs while standing, and finally practice the whole.

Health benefits

1. Swinging your arms, touching your feet and bending your legs help increase the flexibility of the shoulders and legs.

2. Massaging the ribs and the *Dabao* acupoint with your hands and twisting the spine help soothe the liver and activate the spleen.

Step 8 Flying Stance (*Fei Shen Shi*)
Movements

Movement 1: Continue from the previous movement. Shift your weight to the right, bend the left knee and raise it, with calf relaxed and toes pointing down. At the same time, raise your arms slightly above shoulder level, elbows bent slightly, palms facing down and fingertips outward. Inhale with the movement, eyes looking forward (Fig. 119).

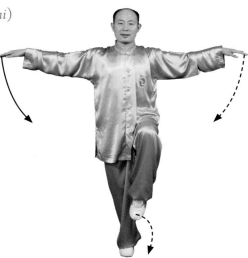

Fig. 119

Movement 2: Bend your right leg and move your left foot 30 degrees forward to the left, toes pointing forward. At the same time, move your arms down and forward to draw an arc, arms naturally down, elbows bent slightly, both arms at navel level, palms facing down, left fingertips forward and to the left, with the right fingertips forward and to the right. Exhale with the movement, eyes looking down and forward (Fig. 120).

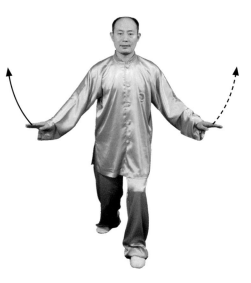

Fig. 120

Movement 3: Shift your weight to the left, straighten and stand on your left leg, bend your right leg and raise it, with your calf free and relaxed and toes pointing down. At the same time, raise your arms, slightly higher than shoulder level, elbows bent slightly, palms facing down. Inhale with the motion, eyes looking forward (Fig. 121).

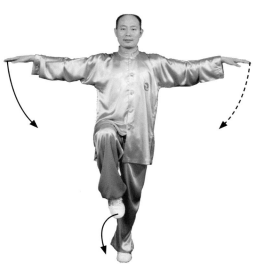

Fig. 121

Movement 4: Bend your left leg and move your right foot forward and 30 degrees to the right, toes pointing forward. At the same time, move your arms down and forward to draw an arc, hands naturally down to reach navel level, elbows bent slightly, palms facing down, left fingertips pointing forward and left and right fingertips forward and pointing right. Exhale with the movement, eyes looking down and forward (Fig. 122).

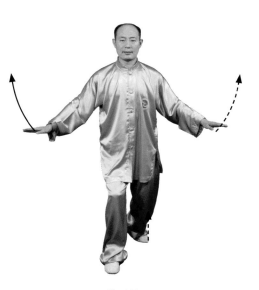

Fig. 122

Movement 5: Repeat Movements 1 to 4, but set the right foot by the inside of the left foot to keep your feet together, knees bent slightly (Figs. 123 and 124).

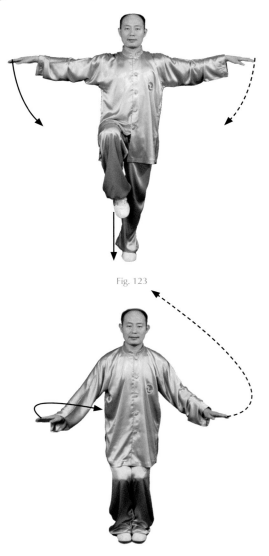

Fig. 123

Fig. 124

Movement 6: Straighten your legs slowly, and move your left arm upward at 45 degrees in an arc; extend it forward at the same time, bending your elbow slightly when the left hand is lifted above the midline, palms down and fingertips up and pointing forward. Move your right arm downward at 45 degrees in an arc and swing it backward, right hand to the midline behind you, elbow bent slightly, palm obliquely up and fingertips pointed down and backward. Inhale with the motion, eyes looking at the raised hand (Fig. 125).

Movement 7: Bend your knees slightly, turn your head to the right and rotate your torso to the right. At the same time, turn the left arm outward and right arm inward, forming an angle of 120 degrees between the forearm and the upper arm, with the left upper

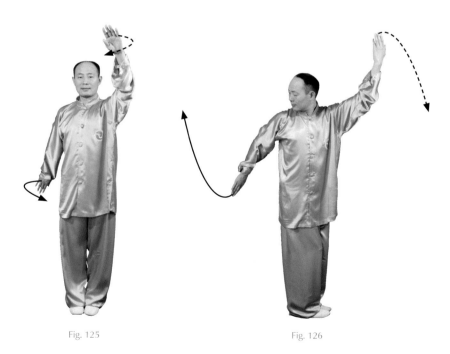

Fig. 125   Fig. 126

arm up 45 degrees above the horizontal line, palm facing outward and fingertips up and pointing forward; the right upper arm extends down at about 45 degrees to the rear, palm facing outward and fingertips down and facing back. Exhale with the movement, with a little pause after, eyes looking down and to the left (Fig. 126).

Movement 8: Straighten your legs slowly, and relax the shoulders and hips to turn the left arm inward and the right arm outward until they are extended horizontally at shoulder height, palms down and fingertips pointing outward. Inhale with the motion, eyes looking forward (Fig. 127).

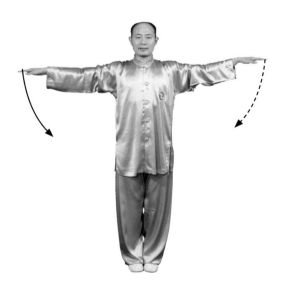

Fig. 127

Movement 9: Bend both knees slightly, relax your shoulders and drop your elbows, then push the palms downward in an arc to waist level, the left palm facing down and slightly forward to the left and the right palm down and forward to the right, fingertips extended. Exhale with the motion, eyes looking down and forward (Fig. 128).

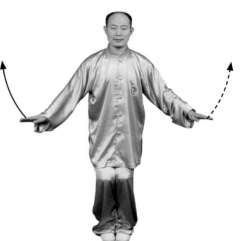

Fig. 128

Movement 10: Repeat Movements 1 to 7, but change the forward step to a backward step. Move your right foot back first (Figs. 129–135).

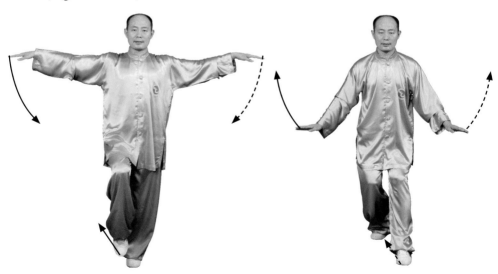

Fig. 129

Fig. 130

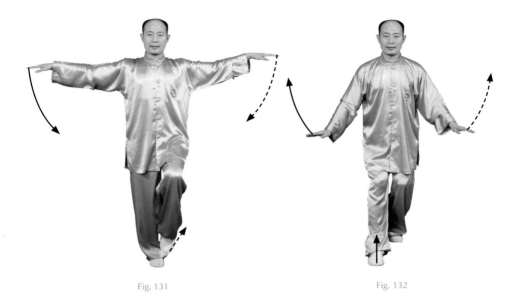

Fig. 131

Fig. 132

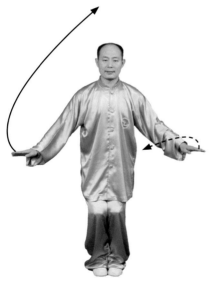

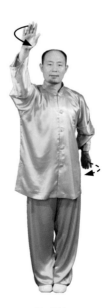

Fig. 133

Fig. 134

Repeat Movement 8, but in the opposite direction, extend both arms horizontally, palms up (Fig. 136).

In this exercise, move four forward steps as one routine and four backward steps for the other.

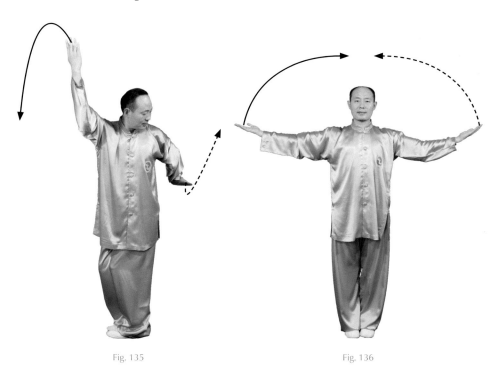

Fig. 135   Fig. 136

Tips

1. When the body rises or drops, or a foot is moved forward or backward, the spinal column twists forward or backward slightly. When arcs are drawn with the arms, the movements should be continuous, relaxed and natural.

2. Don't move your feet after you put them together. When the trunk is rotated fully to the left or right, both arms should be drawn back and forth and pulled up and down and rotated, with the proper degree of relaxation, tightness and coordination.

3. The rotations should be centered around the spine, and your head should turn slowly, eyes level.

4. Turn your head and rotate the spinal column step by step, with the range of the motion changing from small to large.

5. Move forward and backward steadily and breathe with the movement.

6. There is tension in relaxation and relaxation in tension; the shift from one to the other should be slow.

Health benefits

1. Use your arms to effect the rise and fall of *qi* and blood in the body, the movement of the spinal column and its rotation to the right or left draw the meridian channels of the *Sanjiao*, *Ren* and *Du*, and *Dai*, indeed the meridian channels of the whole body, to regulate the *qi* and blood flow in the whole body and prepare for the Ending Stance.

2. Massage the internal organs by moving your chest and abdomen up and down, rotate your spine to stimulate the central nervous system and nerve roots, manipulate the small joints of the spinal column and clear the channels to promote the *qi* and blood flow.

Ending Stance

Movements

Movement 1: Continue from the previous movement. Raise your arms to form a circle above your head, fingertips pointing to each other, 10 cm apart, palms facing obliquely down. Inhale as you raise your arms, eyes looking forward (Fig. 137).

Movement 2: Draw the *qi* back to its origin, move your hands in front of your body and turn your palms inward as you lower your arms slowly to the level of your diaphragm. Palms should be facing down and at navel height, 10 cm apart between the palm and the navel, palms facing the lower *Dantian*, and fingertips pointing obliquely to each other, 5 cm apart. Exhale as you lower your arms, eyes looking down and forward (Fig. 138).

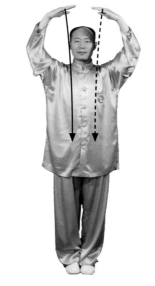

Fig. 137

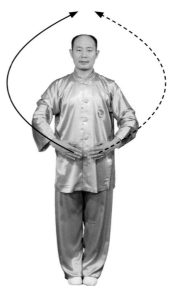

Fig. 138

Moving your hands upward to form a circle and pressing your palms down to the diaphragm make up one routine. Practice the routine three times.

Continue from the end of the third repetition (Fig. 139). Relax both arms and drop them naturally, both palms against the outer thighs. Breathe naturally, eyes looking forward (Fig. 140).

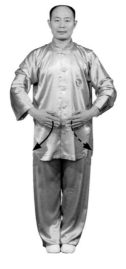

Fig. 139

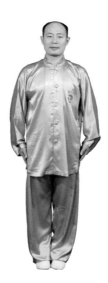

Fig. 140

Tips

1. When moving the arms upward to form the circle and drawing the *qi* back to its origin, use the lower *Dantian* as the center and show internal restraint. Suspend the movement for a brief pause when the palms face the lower *Dantian*.

2. Your movements should be relaxed, soft, natural and fluid. Be calm and relaxed, hold the *qi* and control the mind.

3. After finishing, the practitioner should relax by rubbing the hands, washing the face, clicking the teeth, sounding the celestial drum, rubbing the abdomen, and patting the body.

4. Drink some water after finishing the exercise.

Health benefits

Relax your mind and draw the *qi* back to its origin.

Acupuncture Points

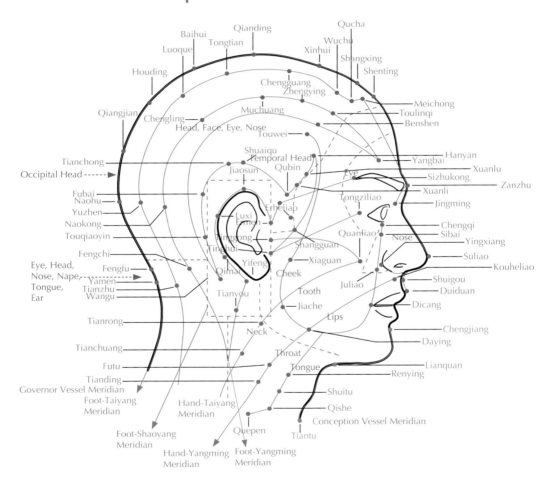

Acupoints on the head and face

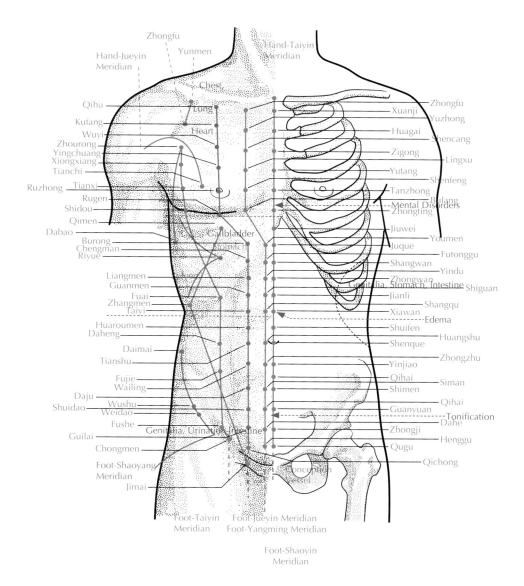

Acupoints on the chest and abdomen

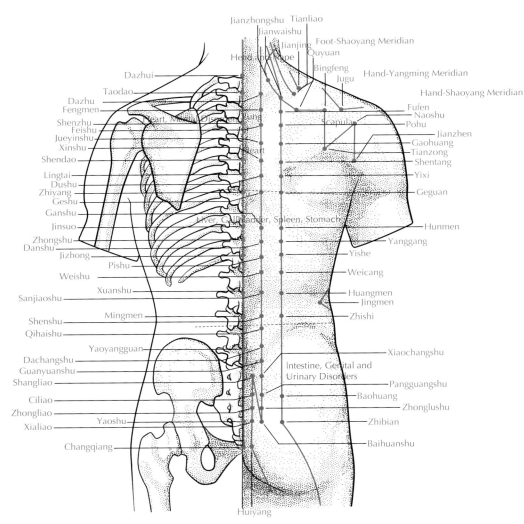

Acupoints on the back and lumbar region

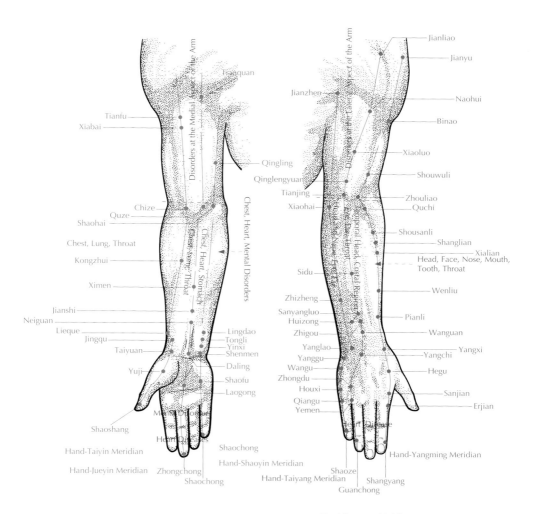

Acupoints in the upper limbs

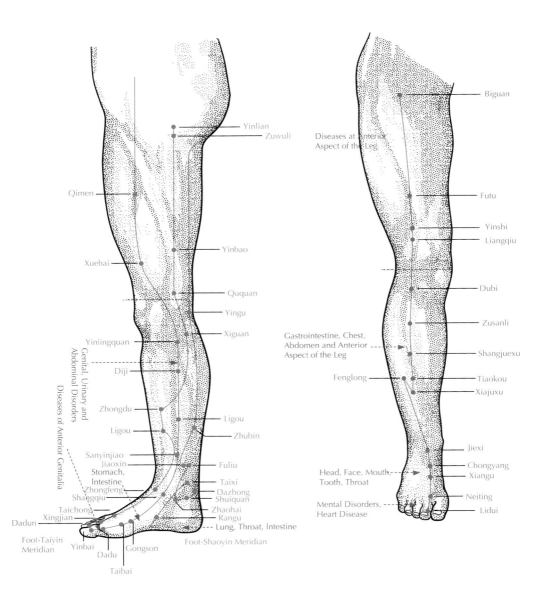

Acupoints in the lower limbs

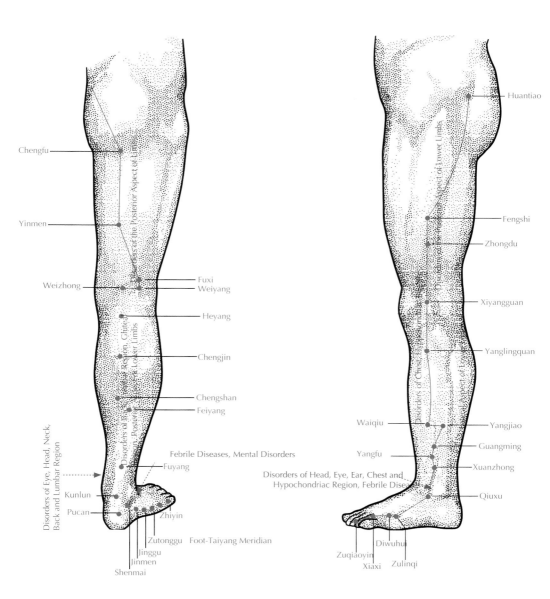

Chengfu

Yinmen

Weizhong

Fuxi
Weiyang

Heyang

Chengjin

Chengshan
Feiyang

Febrile Diseases, Mental Disorders

Fuyang

Disorders of Eye, Head, Neck, Back and Lumbar Region

Kunlun
Pucan
Zhiyin

Zutonggu
Jinggu
Jinmen
Shenmai

Foot-Taiyang Meridian

Disorders of the Posterior Aspect of Limbs

Disorders of Back, Buttock Region, Gluteal Region, Posterior Back of Lower Limbs

Huantiao

Fengshi
Zhongdu

Xiyangguan

Yanglingquan

Waiqiu
Yangfu

Disorders of Head, Eye, Ear, Chest and Hypochondriac Region, Febrile Dise

Yangjiao
Guangming
Xuanzhong
Qiuxu

Zuqiaoyin
Xiaxi
Diwuhui
Zulinqi

Disorders of the Lateral Aspect of Lower Limbs

Disorders of Chest and Hypochondriac

Foot-Shaoyang Meridian of

Acupoints in the lower limbs